Get Lean Gluten Free Cookbook

40+ Fresh & Simple Recipes to KEEP You Lean, Fit & Healthy

Get Lean Gluten Free Cookbook

40+ Fresh & Simple Recipes to KEEP You Lean, Fit & Healthy

Kim Maes, CNC AADP & Jeremy Scott

Get Lean Gluten Free Cookbook

**40+ Fresh & Simple Recipes to KEEP You
Lean, Fit & Healthy**

Authors: Kim Maes, CNC AADP & Jeremy Scott

ISBN-13: 978-1511862226 (CreateSpace Assigned)

Kim Maes: www.cookitallergyfree.com
Jeremy Scott: www.jeremyscottfitness.com

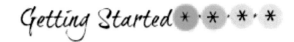

9 TIPS TO GO GLUTEN-FREE, GET LEAN, AND STAY THAT WAY

Eating a gluten-free, clean, fresh, and healthy diet will go a long way in helping you boost your metabolism, loose weight, get super lean, and put you on the path to the healthiest you have ever been. BUT, it only works if you follow some key strategies:

1. **Ditch the Word "Diet"... The "D" Word ONLY equates to Short Term Success.** Instead of considering this to be a diet, consider it as a life-long change. Make it a Lifestyle Change for Permanent Results.

2. **Ditch as many grains as possible.** Don't just replace Gluten-filled baked goods with Gluten-free options. Store-bought gluten-free breads, crackers, muffins, and snacks are usually filled with starchy carbohydrates that will only spike insulin levels and add a nice puffy layer of padding around your middle.

Aim for using either high-protein flours such as coconut flour, almond flour, teff flour, quinoa flour, <u>oat flour</u>, or millet flour if you are going to do any baked goods.

3. **Learn how to read labels.** Gluten can be lurking in surprising places. **Get your gluten-free cheat sheet** and keep it with you so you do not end up getting glutened without knowing it.

4. **Begin a love affair with the perimeter of your grocery store.** This is the easiest way to go gluten-free and become a lean machine. Fruits, vegetables, seafood, lean meats, poultry, nuts and seeds are all naturally gluten free.

5. **While you are in the middle of that love affair with the exterior of your store, include the spice aisle into the mix and make it a threesome.** Getting creative with your spices and herbs can take a bland meal and turn it into a delicious masterpiece.

6. **Plan your meals out at the beginning of the week.** Keep your **Get-Lean Menu Plan and Shopping List** Handy then get everything you need at the beginning of the week so it is all on hand and ready to go.

7. **Challenge yourself to eliminate packaged foods from your pantry.** Eat ONLY whole fresh foods with simple ingredients.

8. Focus on taking care of your gut...from the inside-out. Healing the gut and taking care of your digestion will go a long way in giving you that flat sculpted belly you have been longing for. Probiotic rich foods and probiotic supplements are one way to go about this.

9. Keep Those Meals Simple. Keep your meal ingredients to a minimum. Create fresh and easy meals that only take minutes to throw together. This goes a long way to keeping you on track and helping you from falling off the wagon because it is getting "too hard" or because it takes "too long" to make something. Some of the simplest meals can look and feel the most gourmet when all you are using are fresh wholesome ingredients. The recipes in this cookbook are just that. They will get you in and out of the kitchen fast and you will end up with an amazing meal.

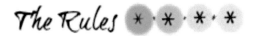

These are your "No's" to live by for the Next 10 Days

1. No Alcohol
2. No Refined Flour Products (bread, bagels, crackers, cake, wraps)
3. No Dairy (yogurt, cheese, milk, ice cream)
4. No Protein or Energy Bars
5. No Desserts or Candy (chocolate bars, ice cream, candy, cookies)
6. No Deli Meats or Processed Meats with Nitrites or Breading
7. No Diet Foods or Beverages
8. No Pre-packaged Microwave Meals or Snack Foods
9. No Foods with Artificial Colors or Flavors
10. No Soy or Soybean Oil

Avoid these Bloating Foods for the Next 10 Days:

1. Brussels Sprouts, Cabbage, Broccoli, Cauliflower, Sugar Snap Peas
2. Inulin, FOS (fructo-oligosaccharides)
3. Onions, Garlic, Mushrooms (in excess)
4. Dried Fruit
5. Beans (in excess)
6. Apples, Apricots, and Cherries
7. Artificial Sweeteners: sorbitol, mannitol, xylitol, isomalt
8. Fructose, High Fructose Corn Syrup

Include these Cleansing Foods:

1. Fresh vegetables and greens (especially celery, cucumber, parsley, asparagus, chard, and kale)
2. Fresh fruit (especially kiwi, pineapple, lemon, grapefruit and organic berries)

Feed Your Body These Fat-Burning Foods:

1. Free-Range/Organic/Antibiotic-Free Poultry, Beef, Pork, Bison, Turkey, Pastured Omega-Eggs
2. Wild Salmon, Trout, Sardines (canned is ok too)
3. Unsweetened Almond Milk, Coconut Milk, or Hemp Milk
4. Nuts and Seeds (unsalted, unsweetened)- Limit each serving to a small handful
5. Coconut Oil, Olive Oil, and Omega-3 EFA's/Fish Oil

Drink Mostly These Beverages:

1. Filtered Water with Fresh Lemon
2. Green or White Tea
3. Sparkling Seltzer- no artificial flavors (e.g. La Croix)

Recommended Dietary Supplements:

1. Daily Essential Multi-Vitamin
2. Protein Powder
3. Powdered Greens
4. Quality Probiotics
5. Quality Omega-3 Fish Oil
6. Vitamin D3

USE CODE: GETLEAN30 for 30% OFF to Stock Up on the above supplements at Olympian Labs

Allowed High-Carb Carbohydrates: *Limit portions of each item to the size of your fist:*

- Sprouted Gluten-Free Grain Breads & Wraps
- Whole Grains: Brown & Wild Rice, Quinoa, Millet, Gluten-Free Oats
- Sweet Potatoes & Yams
- Winter Squash & Turnips, and Peas
- Any Fruit, Fruit Spreads/Jams (unsweetened)
- Beans/Legumes (in moderation), Hummus (also counts as high-fat protein)

Allowed Low-Carb Carbohydrates: *Consume at least a fist-sized portion of each item below:*

- Vegetables & Leafy Greens (i.e., asparagus, green beans, spinach, cucumber, celery, peppers, kale, chard)
- Organic Mixed Berries (i.e., blueberries, strawberries, blackberries, raspberries – frozen or fresh)
- Unsweetened Almond Milk (contains some fat)

Allowed Low-Fat Proteins: *Consume at least a fist-sized portion of each item below:*

- Whole Omega-3 Eggs (2-3 for snacks, 3-6 for meals), Egg Whites
- Lean Beef (Eye of Round, Top Round), Bison, Pork (Tenderloin), Chicken, Turkey
- Lean Bison, Turkey or Chicken Sausage
- White Fish (Cod), Light Tuna, Fresh Seafood (Mussels)
- Stevia-Sweetened Whey Protein, Pea, Hemp Protein

Allowed High-Fat Proteins: *Consume at least a fist-sized portion of each item below:*

- Omega-3 Eggs (3-6 at a time based on size and gender)
- Salmon, Trout
- Canned Sardines, Oysters, Mussels
- Higher Fat Beef (Brisket, Sirloin), Pork (Chop)
- Uncured Pork Bacon
- Uncured Pork, Wild Boar, or Deer Sausage
- Hummus

Allowed Fats: *Limit all oils to 1/2 to 1 Tablespoon, nuts/seeds to a small handful, and nut butters to 1-2 TBSP.*

- Nuts & Seeds (unsalted, unsweetened), Natural Nut Butters (low in salt, unsweetened)
- Olives, Extra Virgin Olive Oil, Olive Oil Mayonnaise
- Avocados, Natural Guacamole
- Coconut Oil, Unsweetened Coconut/Hemp/Almond Milk
- Hemp Oil, Canola Oil, Sesame Oil
- Ground Flax Seeds, Flax Oil

Get Lean, Gluten-Free Meal Plan Template ✳ ✳ ✳ ✳

Day 1, 4, 7, 10 No Carb High Fat	Day 2, 5, 8 Low Carbohydrate Medium Fat	Day 3, 6, 9 Medium Carb/ Medium Fat
Breakfast: Low-Carb Carbohydrate + High-Fat Protein + Fat **Snack:** Fat + Protein **Lunch:** Low-Carb Carbohydrate + High-Fat Protein + Fat **Snack:** Low-Fat Protein + Fat **Dinner:** Low-Carb Carbohydrate + Low-Fat Protein + Fat **Post-workout:** 1-2 Scoops <u>Protein</u> **Drink throughout the day:** Tea, Water, Lemon Water, or Seltzer, black coffee	**Breakfast:** Low-Carb Carbohydrate + Low-Fat Protein + Fat **Snack:** Low-Carb Carbohydrate + High-Fat Protein **Lunch:** Low-Carb Carbohydrate + High-Fat Protein **Snack:** High-Carb Carbohydrate + Low-Fat Protein + Fat **Dinner:** Low-Carb Carbohydrate + Low-Fat Protein + Fat **Post-workout:** 1-2 scoops <u>Protein</u> + Low-Carb Carbohydrate **Drink throughout the day:** Tea, Water, Lemon Water, or Seltzer, black coffee	**Breakfast:** High-Carb Carbohydrate + Low-Carb Carbohydrate + Low-Fat Protein + Fat **Snack:** Low-Carb Carbohydrate + Low-Fat Protein + Fat **Lunch:** Low-Carb Carbohydrate + Low-Fat Protein + Fat **Snack:** Low-Carb Carbohydrate + Low-Fat Protein **Dinner:** High-Carb Carbohydrate + Low-Fat Protein + Fat **Post-workout:** 1-2 scoops <u>Protein</u> **Drink throughout the day:** Tea, Water, Lemon Water, or Seltzer, black coffee

Note: Only follow post-workout nutrition if you exercise that day

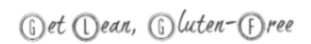 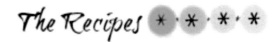

Over 40 Easy and Amazing Gluten-Free Recipes that Will Have you out of the kitchen fast and will keep you lean and healthy for good.

The get lean, gluten-free recipe guide is based on the following rules and the meal plan template. Use the recipes as a base and get creative and you will be able to use this 10-day plan over and over without ever growing bored.

Get lean and stay that way for good!

CONTENTS:

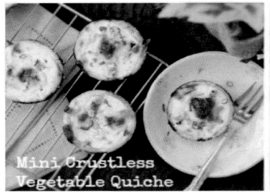

Mini Crustless Vegetable Quiche

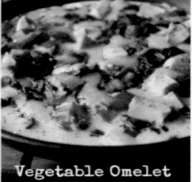

Vegetable Omelet

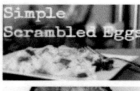

Simple Scrambled Eggs

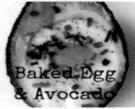

Baked Egg & Avocado

MINI CRUST-LESS VEGETABLE QUICHE

Serves 2-3
Ingredients:
- 1 cup Frozen or Fresh Spinach, Chopped
- 8 eggs
- ¼ cup Plain Coconut Milk
- ½ cup Diced Tomato
- ¼ teaspoon each Salt and Pepper
- ¼ teaspoon Paprika
- 4 slices Cooked and Crumbled Bacon

Directions:
1. Preheat oven to 375F. 2. Arrange spinach on the bottoms of a paper lined muffin pan (approximately 1 tablespoon per cup). 3. Add a thin layer of diced tomato to each cup. Season with salt and pepper. Beat eggs with milk in small bowl with additional salt and pepper. 4. Spoon egg mix into each cup; fill almost to the top. Sprinkle paprika and bacon over top. 5. Bake for 15-20 minutes (check at 15 minutes–you may need less or more time). Save any extras for other mornings.

BAKED EGGS IN AVOCADO

Serves 2
Ingredients:
- 2 ripe avocados
- 4 fresh eggs
- 1/8 teaspoon pepper
- 3 tablespoons bacon, cooked and crumbled

Directions:
1. Preheat the oven to 425 degrees. Slice avocados in half, and remove pit. Scoop out two tablespoons of flesh from the center of avocado, just enough so egg will fit snugly in the center. 2. Place avocado halves in small baking dish. Crack an egg into each avocado half. Crack yolk in first, then let egg whites fill up rest of the shell. Place in oven and bake for 15 to 20 minutes. Cooking time will depend on size of your eggs and avocados. Make sure the egg whites have enough time to set. Top with crumbled bacon. Serve.

SIMPLE SCRAMBLED EGGS WITH HERBS AND VEGETABLES

Serves 2
Ingredients:

- 1 tablespoon coconut oil
- 6 eggs
- 2 tablespoons of water
- Sea salt and freshly ground black pepper
- 3/4 cup chopped mixed fresh herbs (such as parsley and tarragon) and diced red peppers and spinach

Directions:

1. Heat oil in a large nonstick skillet over medium heat.
2. Sautee peppers and spinach for 2 minutes in oil
3. Meanwhile, in a large bowl, whisk together the eggs, water, 1 teaspoon kosher salt, and 1/4 teaspoon pepper.
4. Pour into the pan over peppers and spinach and cook, stirring occasionally, to desired doneness, 4 to 5 minutes. Fold in herbs and serve. Save extras for another morning.

FRESH VEGETABLE OMELET

Serves 2
Ingredients:

- 1 tablespoon coconut oil
- 4 eggs, beaten
- salt and pepper to taste
- 1 red or yellow bell bepper, chopped
- 1 tomato, chopped
- 1 cup chopped spinach or kale
- 1/2 tsp garlic powder (optional)

Directions:

1. In large skillet, sautee the peppers and tomatoes in coconut oil for 3 minutes. Add spinach or kale and sautee for 1 minute longer. Set cooked veggies aside.
2. In another skillet, heat 1 tablespoon of coconut oil and then pour in beaten egg mixture. Sprinkle with salt, pepper, and garlic powder.
3. Allow to cook until the bottom of the eggs are lightly golden brown, then flip and add cooked vegetable mixture into center. Fold egg base in half and cook for a few more minutes. Serve.

OTHER ACCEPTABLE BREAKFAST IDEAS FOR DAYS 1, 4, 7, AND 10:

- **Chicken Sausage and Fresh Spinach, sautéed**
- **Rotisserie Chicken Breast with Avocado and Salsa**
- **Leftover Meat and Vegetables from previous dinner**
- **Hard Boiled Eggs with Salsa and a side of Bacon**
- **Smoked Salmon with Avocado**
- **Deviled Eggs with Avocado or Guacamole**

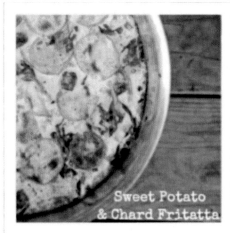
Sweet Potato & Chard Fritatta

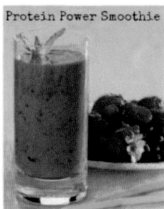
Protein Power Smoothie

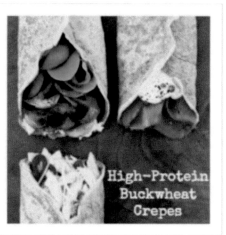
High-Protein Buckwheat Crepes

SWEET POTATO AND SWISS CHARD FRITTATA

Serves 4
Ingredients:

- 3 tablespoons coconut oil
- ½ sweet onion, finely chopped
- 1 small sweet potato *(sliced into VERY thin rounds)*
- 1 bunch Swiss chard *(stem removed, chopped coarsely)*
- 1 dozen eggs
- 1/2 cup coconut milk *(unsweetened)*
- ½ teaspoon sea salt
- ¼ teaspoon black pepper *(to taste)*

Directions:

1. Heat coconut oil in skillet over medium heat. Sautee chopped onion for 3 minutes. Add thin sweet potato rounds and cook for 5 more minutes.
2. Add coarsely chopped Swiss chard into the skillet and continue to cook until the Swiss chard wilts and the potatoes are tender when pierced by a fork.
3. Beat one dozen pastured eggs with coconut milk until the mixture becomes uniform. Add sea salt and black pepper.
4. Reduce the flame to medium-low then pour the beaten eggs and cream into the skillet, over the vegetables. Cook over medium-low until barely set, about six minutes or so.
5. Place the frittata in your oven, under the broiler for about six minutes until it is cooked through. Serve.

PROTEIN POWER SMOOTHIE

Serves 1
Ingredients:

- ½ cup frozen Blueberries
- ½ cup frozen Blackberries
- 1 cup unsweetened vanilla almond milk
- 1 scoop Vanilla Protein Powder
- 1 scoop Powdered Greens

Directions:
Simply blend and serve.
Change up your fruit with other berries, pineapple, peaches or mangoes. Feel free to add fresh greens as well.
Can add 1-2 tablespoons Chia Seeds for additional omega 3's.

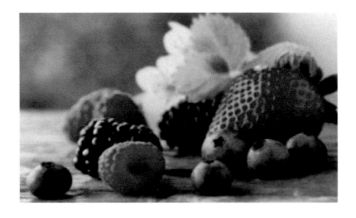

HIGH-PROTEIN BUCKWHEAT CREPES

Serves 2
Ingredients:

- 1 cup Almond Milk, Unsweetened
- ½ cup Cottage Cheese (or additional ½ cup Almond Milk for Dairy-Free version)
- ½ teaspoon Sea Salt
- 2 Large Eggs
- 2 Egg Whites
- 1 ¼ cup Buckwheat Flour
- 2 tablespoons Coconut Oil, in liquid form
- Coconut Oil for cooking
- 6 eggs, scrambled *(for filling)*
- ½ cup red or yellow bell pepper, lightly sautéed in coconut oil for 5 minutes *(for filling)*
- 1 cup Spinach, lightly sautéed in coconut oil for 2 minutes *(for filling)*

Directions:

1. In blender, add Almond Milk, Cottage Cheese (or additional Almond Milk), Sea Salt, Eggs and Egg white. Blend on high for 45 seconds. Add Buckwheat flour and blend another 10 seconds. Refrigerate mixture in blender container for 45 minutes before using.
2. After 45 minutes, remove container, add Coconut Oil (in liquid form) and blend right away before it can solidify in the cold batter.
3. Heat your nonstick skillet over medium heat, just barely enough to make the batter slightly sizzle. Do not let pan get to hot or batter will not spread. Watch how first crepe spreads. You may need to decrease or increase heat.
4. Add ¼ cup batter to the pan and swirl pan to distribute it evenly in a thin layer across the bottom. Cook just until the bottom is browned and can easily be flipped. Cook other side for about 20-30 seconds. Save extra crepes by using wax paper to separate each. Freeze for later.

OTHER ACCEPTABLE BREAKFAST IDEAS FOR DAYS: 2, 5, AND 8

- **Egg Salad made with Olive Oil Mayonnaise and served with Fresh Berries**
- **Leftover Steak mixed into Scrambled eggs and served with Fresh Berries**
- **Variations of the Protein-Packed Smoothie Recipe**
- **Cooked Salmon served with Avocados and Pineapple**
- **Ham and Eggs served with Kiwi or Pineapple**
- **Turkey Breakfast Sausage Links served with Hard-Boiled Eggs and Strawberries**

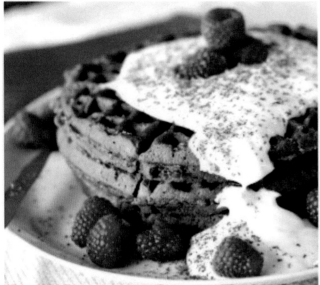

High Protein Cocoa Waffles

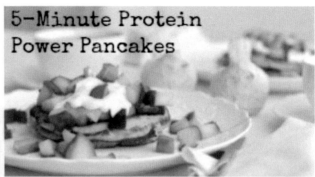

5-Minute Protein Power Pancakes

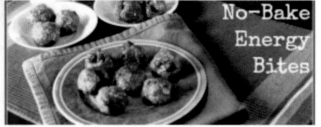

No-Bake Energy Bites

HIGH-PROTEIN COCOA WAFFLES

Serves 2-4
Ingredients:

- 1 cup almond flour
- 1 scoop vanilla protein powder
- ¼ cup unsweetened cocoa powder
- 1 ½ teaspoon baking powder
- 1/2 teaspoon xanthan gum
- ¼ teaspoon salt
- 3 eggs, separated
- 2 tablespoons coconut oil
- 1/2 cup coconut milk, unsweetened
- 1 teaspoon vanilla extract

Directions:

1. Mix almond flour, protein powder, cocoa powder, xanthan gum, baking powder, and salt in one bowl. **2.** In another bowl, add egg yolks, coconut oil, coconut milk, and vanilla and mix well. **3.** Fold wet ingredients into dry ingredients. **4.** With electric mixer, beat egg whites in small bowl until slightly stiff. Then gently fold into mixed batter. **5.** Pour batter into greased pre-heated waffle iron (following instructions on your waffle iron). Can also be made as pancakes if desired by adding an additional ½ cup coconut milk to batter.

5-MINUTE PROTEIN POWER PANCAKES

Serves 4-6
Ingredients:
- 1 ripe Banana
- 3 Eggs
- 2 Egg Whites
- 1 cup Almond Milk, unsweetened
- 1 Tbsp Vanilla Extract
- 2 ¼ cup blanched Almond Flour
- 1 Scoop Vanilla Protein Powder
- 2 tsp Baking Soda
- ¼ tsp Salt
- 1 Tbsp Coconut Oil for cooking

Directions:
1. In your food processor or high-speed blender, blend together banana, eggs, egg whites, and Almond Milk until smooth. Add almond flour, protein powder, baking soda, and salt.
2. Heat some of the Coconut Oil in large skillet, and add batter to make 3-4 inch diameter pancakes. Cook about 3 minutes until golden on bottom and pancake wants to flip easily (when bubbles start to appear and pop). Feel free to add blueberries or other fruit to pancakes before flipping, if desired. **3.** Flip and cook 2 minutes longer. Add more oil as necessary.

BREAKFAST TIPS:
- **Make big batches of your high-protein crepes, pancakes, waffles, and mini quiches on the weekends, or whenever you have extra time to spend in the kitchen. They all freeze wonderfully and will be perfect to just grab and warm quickly on your busy mornings.**
- **Energy Bites are also great to grab as snacks as well and will last over a week in the refrigerator.**
- **Make a batch of Hard-Boiled Eggs to keep ready you need something quick on the go. Pair with an energy-bite or fresh berries.**

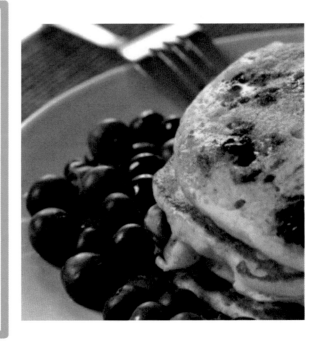

NO-BAKE HIGH-PROTEIN ENERGY BITES

Makes 20-28
Ingredients:

- 1 Cup Certified Gluten Free Oats
- 3 Tbsp Ground Chia Seeds
- 3 Tbsp Hemp Seeds
- 2 Tbsp Raw Cacao Powder
- 3/4 Scoop Vanilla Protein Powder
- 1 tsp Cinnamon
- 1/4 tsp Sea Salt
- 2/3 Cup Almond Butter
- 2 Tbsp Maple Syrup or Raw Honey
- 2 tsp Vanilla
- *Optional*: Can mix in 1/3 cup of dried cherries, or chopped pumpkin seeds, or mini chocolate chips

Directions:

1. In large bowl, combine Oats, Ground Chia, Hemp Seeds, Cacao Powder, Protein Powder, Cinnamon, and Sea Salt. Add in Almond Butter, Maple Syrup, Vanilla, and optional Mix-Ins, if using. Mix until just combined. **2.** Scoop 1 Tablespoon of mixture and roll between hands into ball. Place on cookie sheet. Repeat until all the mixture is used. Depending on the size, this should make about 20-28.
3. Place cookie sheet in refrigerator for about 30 minutes to set. Once chilled, store in airtight container in refrigerator for up to 1 week. Pair with Hard-Boiled Eggs as a great grab-and-go meal.

OTHER ACCEPTABLE BREAKFAST IDEAS FOR DAYS: 3, 6, 9

- **Scrambled Eggs with Salsa and Sweet Potato Hash Browns**
- **Steel-Cut Oats with Peaches and (Coconut) Cream**
- **Chicken Breakfast Sausage with Roasted Peppers and Roasted Sweet Potatoes**
- **Steak, Sweet Potato, Red Pepper Hash**
- **High-Protein Pancake PB&J "Sandwiches"- Sandwich fresh berries and 1 Tablespoon Nut Butter between two High-Protein Power Pancakes**

SNACK IDEAS FOR DAYS 1, 4, 7, & 10

Pick from these 2 times per day:
- 1 Can of Light Tuna in Water mixed with Olive Oil Mayonnaise on Cucumber Slices
- Handful of Cashews and Walnuts
- Pumpkin Seeds and Raw Carrots
- Sliced Hard-Boiled eggs on Cucumber Slices
- Peanut Butter or Almond Butter on Celery Sticks
- Celery Sticks filled with 1 Can of Light Tuna mixed with Olive Oil Mayonnaise
- Handful of Almonds with ¼ Avocado

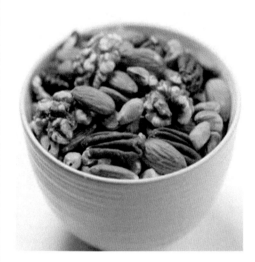

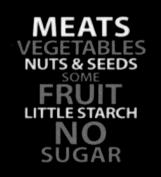

MEATS
VEGETABLES
NUTS & SEEDS
SOME
FRUIT
LITTLE STARCH
NO
SUGAR

SNACK IDEAS FOR DAYS 2, 5, & 8:

Pick from these 2 times per day:
- Hard-Boiled Egg and Berries or Peaches
- Gluten-Free Organic Beef Jerky with Carrots
- Kale Chips (recipe follows) with Almonds
- Pumpkin Seeds and Cucumber Slices
- Organic Hummus with Carrot, Celery, and Cucumber Slices
- Handful of Pistachios and two kiwi fruit
- Homemade Trail Mix (recipe follows)

SNACK IDEAS FOR DAYS 3, 6, & 9

Pick from these 2 times per day:
- High-Protein Banana Muffins (recipe follows)
- High-Protein Raspberry Coconut Muffins (recipe follows)
- No-Bake Energy Bites (Recipe under Breakfasts)
- 1 High-Protein Granola Bars (recipe follows)
- Turkey Slices with Zucchini Sticks and Cucumber Slices
- Almond Milk mixed with Prograde Lean

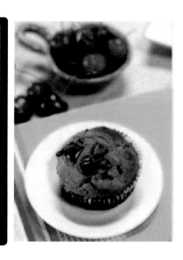

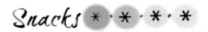

EASY CRISPY KALE CHIPS

Heat oven to 375 Degrees F. Remove stems and roughly chop **two bunches of kale**. Toss with 2 tablespoons **coconut oil**, 1 teaspoon **minced garlic**, ½ teaspoon **garlic salt**, ½ teaspoon **Sea Salt**, and ½ teaspoon **Smoked Paprika**. Spread evenly and spaced out on baking sheet. Cook for 8 minutes and stir once. Cook for 2-4 minutes more, until edges become slightly brown and leaves are crispy.

HIGH-ENERGY GRANOLA BARS

Makes 24 Medium-Sized Bars
Ingredients:
- 1 cup Certified Gluten Free Oats1 cup Quinoa Flakes
- 2/3 cup Almond Flour
- 2 Scoops Vanilla Protein Powder
- 1/4 cup Ground Chia Seeds
- 2 teaspoon Ground Cinnamon
- 3/4 teaspoon Sea Salt, fine
- ½ Cup Pumpkin Seeds
- 1/4 cup Dark Chocolate pieces – Optional
- 2 eggs, beaten
- 1 egg white, beaten
- 1/2 cup Cold-Pressed Unrefined Coconut Oil
- 1/3 cup Honey
- 1 tablespoon Vanilla

Directions:
1. Preheat oven to 350 degrees. Lightly grease a 9x13 inch glass-baking pan.
2. Sift together in large bowl: Gluten Free Oats, Quinoa Flakes, Almond Flour, Protein Powder, Ground Chia (or hemp) Seeds, Cinnamon, Sea Salt, Pumpkin Seeds, and Dark Chocolate.
3. Make small well in center of dry mixture. Add: beaten eggs, egg whites, coconut oil, honey, and vanilla.
4. Squish/mix together with hands. Press into prepared baking dish. You do not have to press all the way to edges (will not spread while baking) if you want a thicker and chewier bar.
5. Bake for about 30 minutes, or until edges look slightly golden.

HIGH-PROTEIN BANANA MUFFINS

Makes 10 Muffins
Ingredients:
- 1 cup natural peanut or almond butter
- 3 large eggs
- 1 scoop Vanilla Protein Powder
- 2 medium sized very ripe banana
- 3/4 teaspoon baking soda
- 2 teaspoons vanilla
- 2 tablespoons honey (optional)
- Mix-ins of choice: mini chocolate chips, shredded coconut, raisins, cranberries

Directions:
1. Preheat oven to 400 degrees F.
2. Place all ingredients into a blender; blend until well mixed like the consistency of a thick smoothie.
3. Pour batter into muffin liners in pan. Use a rubber scraper to remove the last bit from the blender.
4. Add mix-ins of choice to each muffin and lightly stir into each cup with toothpick.
5. Cook for 12- 15 minutes for full size muffins and 8-10 minutes for mini muffins. Freeze extras for quick grab and go snacks.

EAT CLEAN

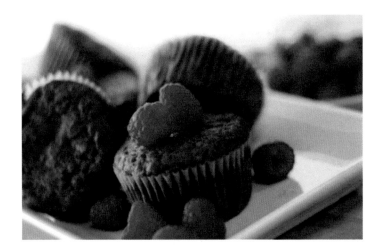

HIGH-PROTEIN RASPBERRY COCONUT MUFFINS

Makes 16-18 Muffins
Ingredients:

- 6 large eggs
- 1/3 cup coconut milk
- ¼ cup honey or maple syrup
- 2 teaspoons vanilla extract
- 8 tablespoons coconut oil, melted
- ¾ cup coconut flour
- 2 tablespoons vanilla protein powder
- 2 teaspoons baking powder
- 1 teaspoon baking soda
- ¾ teaspoon sea salt
- ½ cup applesauce
- 1 ½ cup frozen raspberries

Directions:
1. Preheat oven to 375ºF and adjust rack to middle position
2. Line your muffin pan with paper muffin liners
3. Beat eggs with electric stand mixer on medium speed. Add coconut milk, honey, vanilla, almond extract and coconut oil.
4. Mix coconut flour, baking powder, baking soda, and salt in a medium bowl Slowly add in dry ingredients and mix on low speed only until just combined and lumps are gone.
5. Fold in applesauce and then very gently fold in raspberries.
6. Spoon batter into muffin cups and bake for 18 minutes, or until lightly brown on top. Store muffins in air-tight container for 2 days on counter. Freeze any remaining muffins.

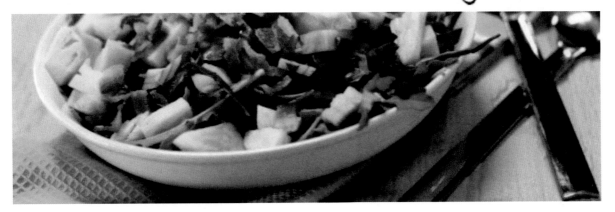

BUILD A BETTER SALAD – PICK FROM EACH BOX & SWITCH IT UP

TIP: Invest in some portable food containers, build your salad in the morning, and then bring the dressing and toss on the go when ready to eat

These are acceptable toppings for Days 1, 4, 7, and 10 of the Get Lean Meal

STEP 1: PICK YOUR GREENS
(No limit to how much)
- Arugula
- Spinach
- Romaine
- Kale, Chard, Collards
- Radicchio
- Mustard Greens

STEP 2: PICK YOUR PROTEIN(S)
(About ½ - 1 Cup)
- Chicken or Turkey
- Shrimp or Crab
- Tuna
- Salmon
- Steak
- Hard-Boiled Eggs
- Bacon

PICK YOUR SUPERFOOD TOPPINGS:
(No limit)
- Bell Peppers
- Tomatoes
- Avocado (limit to 3 slices)
- Cucumbers
- Carrot
- Celery
- Asparagus

EXTRA TOPPING CHOICES:
(No more than 2 Tablespoons of these)
- Black Olives
- Pine Nuts
- Pistachios
- Almond Slices
- Pumpkin Seeds
- Sunflower Seeds

SIMPLE DRESSING:
Combine 1 Tablespoon Coconut Oil with 2 teaspoons of Apple Cider Vinegar and ¼ teaspoon of Sea Salt. Use on Salads and Roasted Vegetables.

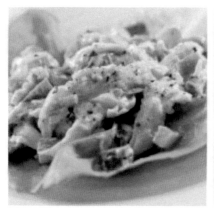 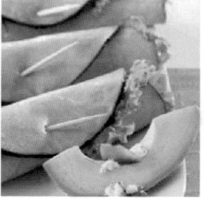 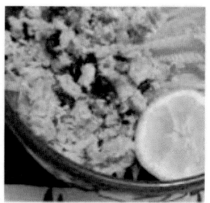

CHICKEN SALAD

Serves 4
Ingredients:

- 1 whole organic rotisserie chicken, or 4-5 large chicken breasts, cooked and cubed
- 1 cup mango, cut in small pieces (or green or red grapes, quartered)
- 3/4 cup organic chopped walnuts
- 3-4 stalks organic celery, cut into small pieces
- 1/4 cup diced red onion
- 2/3 cup organic olive oil mayonnaise
- Juice of ½ a lemon
- 1 teaspoon Sriracha Sauce (or other red chili sauce)
- 1/2 teaspoon organic curry powder
- ½ teaspoon salt and pepper, each

Directions:

1. In large mixing bowl, add chicken pieces, mango pieces, walnuts, celery, red onion and toss.
2. In small bowl, mix together mayonnaise, lemon juice, Sriracha sauce, curry powder, salt and pepper.
3. Pour over chicken mixture and toss well. Serve on lettuce leaves.

CRANBERRY TUNA WRAPS

Serves 4
Ingredients:

- 1/3 cup organic olive oil mayonnaise
- ¼ cup dried cranberries, coarsely chopped
- 1 tablespoon dill, fresh, chopped
- ½ teaspoon sea salt
- ½ teaspoon black pepper, freshly ground
- ¼ teaspoon lemon zest
- 1 teaspoon fresh lemon juice
- 12 ounces water-packed tuna fish, drained
- 8 leaves of Bibb Lettuce (or large Romaine leaves)

Directions:

1. In large mixing bowl, add mayonnaise, cranberries, dill, salt, pepper, lemon zest and juice, and tuna. Combine gently until evenly mixed.
2. Place about ¼ cup of mixture in the middle of each lettuce leaf. Roll and serve.

TURKEY, SPINACH, VEGETABLE AND AVOCADO ROLL-UPS

Serves 2
Ingredients:

2 teaspoons Dijon Mustard
2 teaspoons honey
10 slices turkey breast
2 cups baby spinach
1 avocado, thinly sliced
1/4 large carrot, julienned
1/4 large red pepper, thinly sliced

Directions:

1. In a small bowl mix together the Dijon mustard and honey until well combined.
2. Lay a slice of turkey on a plate or cutting board. Spread a ½ teaspoon of the honey-mustard mixture widthwise along the turkey about 2 inches from the end of the slice.
3. Place a pile of spinach on top of the honey-mustard mixture, top spinach with a couple of slices of avocado, some of the julienned carrot, and a few slices of the red pepper.
4. Roll it all up in the turkey slice. Repeat with remaining turkey slices. Serve.

OTHER ACCEPTABLE LUNCH IDEAS FOR DAYS: 2, 5, AND 8

- **Egg Salad with a side of berries**
- **Spinach Salad with Vegetable, Nuts, and Seeds and Apple Cider Vinegar Dressing**
- **Leftovers from Dinner the night before**
- **Nori Wraps with your favorite meat and veggies**
- **Lettuce "Sandwich" Wraps – see ideas on next page**
- **Mini Egg Quiches leftover from Breakfast**
- **Tuna-Stuffed Deviled Eggs**

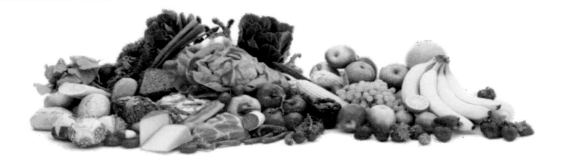

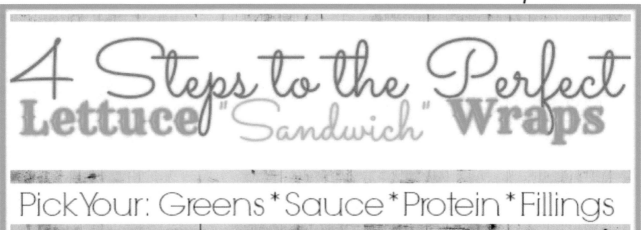

Pick Your: Greens * Sauce * Protein * Fillings

1. PICK YOUR GREENS:

- Cabbage
- Bibb
- Romaine
- Endive
- Large Spinach Leaves
- Kale
- Collards
- Chard

2. PICK YOUR SAUCES/SPICES:

- Mustard
- Olive Oil Mayonnaise
- Pesto
- Guacamole
- Horseradish
- Hummus
- Flavored Mayonnaise
- Hot Sauce
- Sriracha
- Oil and Vinegar
- Ginger
- Lemon Juice

3. PICK YOUR PROTEIN:

- Rotisserie Chicken Pieces
- Turkey Slices
- Roast Beef Slices
- Cooked Shrimp
- Crab or Lobster
- Tuna – Water packed
- Ground Bison, Turkey, or Chicken
- Turkey Bacon
- Grilled or Smoked Salmon
- Diced Hard-Boiled Eggs
- Scrambled Eggs

4. PICK YOUR HERBS AND VEGETABLES:

- Avocado
- Red, Orange, or Yellow Bell Peppers
- Tomatoes
- Red Onions
- Zucchini Ribbons
- Cilantro
- Basil
- Chives
- Fresh Figs
- Sauerkraut
- Pickles or Olives

REMEMBER:

- Clean Eating does not mean giving up your favorite sandwiches.
- Just make a few changes and you can still eat the food you love
- Wrap your favorite fillings in some crispy crunchy lettuce
- Add your favorite seasonings and sauces from the boxes and then wrap it all up like a burrito
- Great to take on the go, to work or school

26

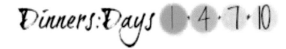

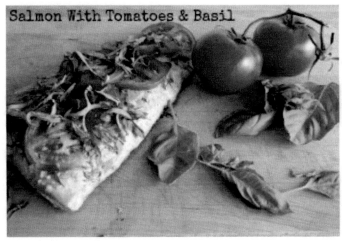

Salmon With Tomatoes & Basil

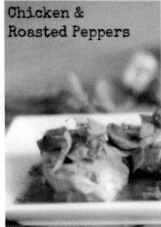

Chicken & Roasted Peppers

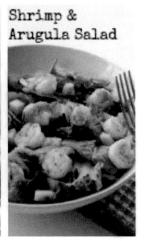

Shrimp & Arugula Salad

WILD SALMON WITH TOMATOES AND BASIL

Serves 4
Ingredients:
- 2 pounds Wild Salmon Fillet
- 3 cloves of garlic, minced
- 3 Tablespoons olive oil
- 1 1/2 teaspoon sea salt, or more to taste, divided
- 1 cup fresh basil, divided 1/2 cup chopped fine; other 1/2 very thinly slivered)
- 2 Roma tomatoes, very thinly sliced

Directions:

1. Preheat your grill to medium high. **2**. In a bowl, mash minced garlic, 1 teaspoon sea salt, and 1/2 cup finely chopped basil with the back of a spoon until you get a nice paste. Then add in the olive oil and blend together. **3**. Lightly oil a heavy piece of aluminum foil that is slightly larger than your salmon fillet. Place salmon on it, skin side down, and spread garlic basil paste over the top of the fish. Then, over paste, layer thinly sliced tomatoes to cover salmon. **4**. Sprinkle with the remaining sea salt and transfer salmon to the grill. Cook about 10 minutes, or until salmon flakes easily with a fork. **5**. When fish is done, slide off foil onto serving plate and top with the reserved slivered basil. Serve with a Spinach Salad topped with raw cucumbers and peppers.

GRILLED CHICKEN BREASTS WITH ROASTED PEPPERS

Serves 2
Ingredients:
- 2 pounds boneless skinless chicken breasts
- 3 Tablespoons Coconut Oil
- ¾ teaspoon each Sea Salt and Pepper
- 1 teaspoon Smoked Paprika
- 2 Red, Yellow, or Orange Bell Peppers, sliced in quarters and seeds removed

Directions:
1. Preheat grill to medium-high heat. 2. Pour Coconut Oil evenly over the Chicken Breasts and Pepper Slices. Season everything evenly with Smoked Paprika, Sea Salt, and Pepper. 3. Place Chicken and Peppers on grill and cook for about 20 minutes, turning once, halfway through. Can serve over chopped romaine lettuce with sliced avocado. Save any left-over chicken to use for lunch the next day.

ROASTED SHRIMP AND ARUGULA CHOPPED SALAD

Serves 2-4
Ingredients:
- 1 bunch fresh asparagus spears, trimmed
- 3 cups arugula, roughly chopped
- 1 pound frozen, peeled and deveined cooked shrimp with tails intact, thawed
- 1 cups cherry tomatoes, halved
- ½ avocado, peeled and sliced
- 1 Tbsp Pine Nuts
- 4 Tbsp light balsamic vinegar dressing
- Sea salt and pepper to taste

Directions:
1. In a large skillet cook asparagus, covered, in a small amount of boiling lightly salted water for 3 minutes or until crisp-tender; drain in colander. Run under cold water until cool. 2. Place asparagus on plates; top with arugula, shrimp, tomatoes, and avocado, and pine nuts. 3. Drizzle with dressing. Sprinkle with sea salt and pepper and serve. Serves 2.

OTHER ACCEPTABLE DINNER IDEAS FOR DAYS 1, 4, 7, AND 10:

- **Bacon Wrapped Chicken with Spinach Salad**
- **Hamburger with no Bun topped with Tomatoes and Avocado**
- **Grilled Steak with Kale and Avocado Salad**
- **Grilled Shrimp with Grilled Zucchini**
- **Baked Cod drizzled with Coconut Oil and Sea Salt and Paprika**
- **Fresh Vegetable Omelet with**
- **Baked Eggs in Avocado**

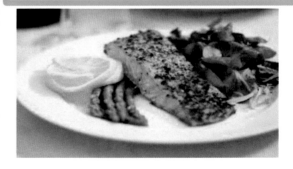

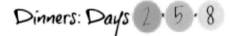

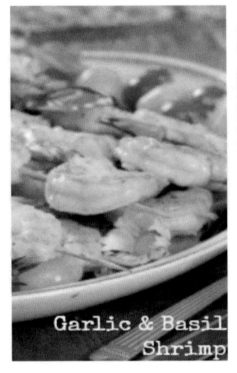

Garlic & Basil
Shrimp

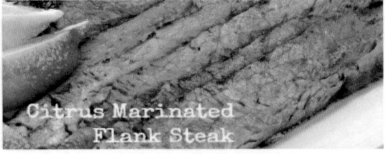

Citrus Marinated
Flank Steak

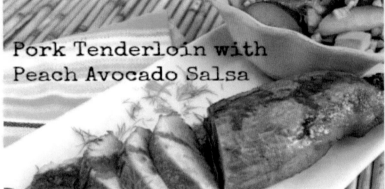

Pork Tenderloin with
Peach Avocado Salsa

GARLIC AND BASIL SHRIMP

Serves: 2-4
Ingredients:

- 2 pounds shrimp (16/20), peeled and deveined, tails on
- 3 tablespoons coconut oil
- 2 teaspoons sugar
- 1 teaspoon smoked paprika
- ½ teaspoon sea salt
- 3 cloves garlic, grated
- 3 tablespoons fresh basil, finely chopped
- 1 lemon, zested

Directions:
1. In a large mixing bowl, combine the shrimp, coconut oil, sugar, smoked paprika, salt, garlic, half of the basil, and lemon zest. Let the shrimp marinate for 20 minutes.
2. Preheat a grill pan or a skillet over high heat.
3. When the pan is hot, grill the shrimp until they are just cooked through and turning pink, about 2 minutes per side. Top with remaining basil and serve immediately with a big spinach salad and a size of quinoa.

FLANK STEAK WITH CITRUS MARINADE

Serves: 2-4
Ingredients:

- 1 2lb Flank Steak (or Skirt Steak)
- 1 orange, juiced
- 1 lime juiced
- 4 cloves garlic, peeled and crushed
- 2 teaspoon brown mustard
- 1 ½ tablespoon Apple Cider Vinegar

Directions:
1. Combine juice of orange and lime, crushed garlic, mustard, and vinegar to bowl and combine. **2**. Place steak in 1 gallon ziplock bag. Pour marinade over steak in bag, seal, and refrigerate for 1-2 hours. **3**. Preheat grill to medium-high heat. Grill steak for 6-7 minutes per side, turning once. **4**. Slice against the grain and serve with grilled asparagus or peppers.

ROASTED PORK TENDERLOIN WITH PEACH AVOCADO SALSA

Serves: 3-4
Ingredients:
- 1 1/2 pound pork tenderloin
- 3/4 cup apple cider vinegar
- 1/4 cup honey
- 1/4 cup white wine
- 1/2 teaspoon sea salt, divided
- 1 Avocado, diced
- 2 peaches, sliced
- 1 red onion, finely chopped
- 2 Tablespoons fresh lime juice

Directions:
1. Preheat oven to 375 degrees. Place pork in a re-sealable ziplock bag. In a bowl, combine balsamic vinegar, honey, white wine, and half of the sea salt. Whisk to combine, then pour mixture over the pork to marinate for about thirty minutes
2. While pork is marinating, combine the avocado, peaches, red onion, juice from lime, and other half of sea salt in a bowl. Set aside.
3. Place pork in a small roasting pan. Pour remaining marinade from bag over pork, then cover pan with foil. Roast for 15 minutes, covered. Then remove foil and roast uncovered for another 5-10 minutes, or until internal temperature is about 140 degrees
4. Slice the pork into thin medallions, pour a little of the salsa over it, then drizzle it all with the reduced balsamic sauce and enjoy!

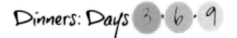
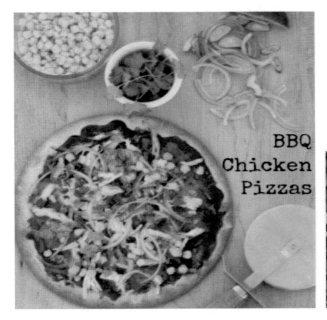
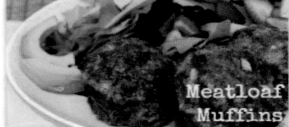
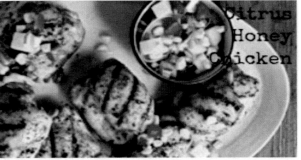

BBQ Chicken Pizzas

Meatloaf Muffins

Citrus Honey Chicken

MEATLOAF MUFFINS WITH BARBEQUE GLAZE

Serves: 4
Ingredients:

- 1/2 cup favorite barbeque sauce
- 1 ½ pounds ground beef or bison (organic, grass-fed, preferably)
- 3 cloves garlic, minced
- 1/2 cup almond milk
- 1 egg
- 1/4 cup celery, finely chopped
- 1/2 cup onion, finely chopped
- 1 1/2 teaspoon salt
- 1/4 teaspoon ground black pepper, or to taste
- 1 cup gluten free cracker crumbs, (such as Glutino crackers or Pretzels crushed into crumbs
- 1-2 tablespoons additional barbeque sauce

Directions:
1. Preheat oven to 350 degrees F. **2.** Place a tablespoon of barbeque sauce in the bottom of each muffin opening. 1 1/2 pounds of meat should make about 9 muffins. **3.** In a bowl, mix thoroughly all remaining ingredients, except for the last 1-2 Tablespoons of Barbeque Sauce. **4.** Press meat mixture on top of the ketchup and sugar, filling each muffin cup to the top. Then with a spoon make a little well in the top of each meat-filled muffin tin and place a small dollop of the Barbeque Sauce in each little well. **5.** Bake in preheated oven for 25-30 minutes or until juices are clear. Serve with cooked quinoa and a salad.

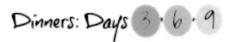

BARBEQUE CHICKEN PIZZAS WITH ALMOND FLOUR PIZZA CRUST

Serves 4

Ingredients:

- 2 Almond Flour Pizza Crusts **(recipe below)**
- 1 tablespoon Olive Oil, divided
- 1/2 cup Barbeque Sauce
- 1 cup leftover shredded Rotisserie Chicken
- ½ of a Red Onion, very thinly sliced
- ¼ cup frozen Corn
- ½ teaspoon Sea Salt
- 3 tablespoons Cilantro, chopped
- Sea Salt to taste.

Directions:

1. Preheat oven to 400 degrees F. Spread barbeque sauce evenly over both crusts. **2.** Top with the shredded chicken, red onion, corn, and sea salt. **3.** Bake for 10 minutes, until crust is just beginning to crisp. **4.** Remove, top with chopped cilantro, and slice. Serve with a big arugula and vegetable salad.

GRAIN-FREE ALMOND FLOUR CRUST

Serves: 2-4

Ingredients:

- 2 cups Almond Meal/Flour
- 2 eggs
- 2 tablespoon extra virgin olive oil
- 1 teaspoon salt

Directions:

1. Preheat oven to 350 degrees. Mix all the ingredients together to form a dough. **2.** Lightly oil two pieces of parchment paper. **3.** Put the dough between the two pieces of parchment paper and roll it until desired thickness. **4.** Move the pizza and bottom piece of parchment paper to a pizza tray. **5.** Bake for 10-15 minutes – until middle is cooked. Take out of the oven and top with favorite toppings.

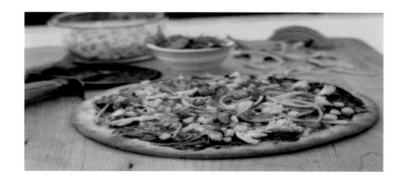

GRILLED CITRUS-HONEY CHICKEN THIGHS

Serves: 2-4
Ingredients:

- 1 cup Freshly Squeezed Orange Juice
- 2 teaspoons Gluten-Free Tamari Soy Sauce, or For Soy-Free: Use Coconut Secrets Raw Coconut Aminos 1 tablespoon honey
- 1/2 tsp minced ginger
- 1/2 tsp crushed garlic
- 1/2 tsp sea salt
- 1/8 tsp roasted red chili paste (optional)
- 2 scallions, roughly chopped
- 1 1/2 - 2 pounds boneless, skinless chicken thighs (preferably Organic and Free-range)

Directions:
1. In medium bowl, create marinade. Whisk together: Orange Juice, Soy Sauce (or Soy-Free option), Honey, Ginger, Garlic, Sea Salt, Chili Paste, and Scallions. **2**. Place Chicken in a glass bowl or baking dish that just fits chicken pieces. Pour Marinade over chicken so all pieces are covered in marinade. Marinade at least 1 hour and up to 8 hours. **3**. Preheat Grill. Remove Chicken from Marinade. Season chicken on both sides generously with Sea Salt and Cracked Pepper. Grill Chicken over medium-high heat for about 9 – 10 minutes per side. Serve with Grilled Peppers or Asparagus.

OTHER ACCEPTABLE DINNER IDEAS FOR DAYS 3, 6, AND 9:

- **Roasted Chicken Breasts with Sweet Potatoes and a side of Cooked Quinoa**
- **Grilled Fish of Choice with Carrots and Parsnips Sauteed in Coconut Oil**
- **Steak and Eggs and a side of Roasted Sweet Potatoes**
- **Baked Salmon with Roasted Beets and some Steamed Asparagus**
- **Grilled Chicken Sausage and Grilled Zucchini Halves brushed with Coconut Oil**
- **Pan-Fried Pork Chops with Sauteed Onions and Apples**
- **Roasted Turkey Breasts with Carrots and Parsnips**

STEPS TO PERFECTLY GRILLED OR ROASTED VEGETABLES:

Prepare and Cook Your Seasoned Vegetables:

ASPARAGUS: Trim off woody ends (about one inch off the bottom). Season with one of the options below. Remove from marinade. **For oven method**: Place on baking sheet and roast in oven preheated to 400 degrees for 8 – 10 minutes, until tender. **For grill method**: Place on foil and cook for about 8 minutes, until tender.

BELL PEPPERS: Cut into ½ inch thick lengthwise pieces and remove seeds. Season with one of the options below. **For oven method**: Place on baking sheet and roast in oven preheated to 400 degrees for 10-12 minutes, until tender. **For grill method:** Place on foil and cook for about 10 minutes, until tender.

CARROTS: Cut into 1 ½ inch pieces on an angle. Season with one of the options below. **For oven method**: Place on baking sheet and roast in oven preheated to 400 degrees for 20 minutes, until tender. **For grill method**: Place on foil and cook for about 15 or so minutes, until tender.

PLUM TOMATOES: Cut in half lengthwise and remove seeds. Season with one of the options below. **For oven method**: Place on baking sheet and roast in oven preheated to 400 degrees for 15 minutes, until tender. **For grill method**: Place on foil, cut side down, and cook for about 10 or so minutes, until tender.

SWEET ONIONS: Cut into ½ inch thick rounds. Season with one of the options below. **For oven method**: Place on baking sheet and roast in oven preheated to 400 degrees for 25 minutes, until tender. **For grill method**: Place on foil and cook for about 20 or so minutes, until tender.

SWEET POTATOES: Dice potatoes into 1 inch pieces. Season with coconut oil, cinnamon, and sea salt. **For oven method**: Place on baking sheet and roast in oven preheated to 400 degrees for 40 minutes, until tender. **For grill method**: Place on foil and cook for about 30 minutes, until tender.

ZUCCHINI: Halve zucchini lengthwise. Season with one of the options below. **For oven method**: Place on baking sheet and roast in oven preheated to 400 degrees for 20 minutes, until tender. **For grill method**: Place on foil, cut side down, and cook for about 15 minutes, until tender.

STEPS TO PERFECTLY GRILLED OR ROASTED VEGETABLES:

Seasoning Options For Your Vegetables

Option 1 - Mix prepared vegetables of choice in a ziplock bag with ¼ Apple Cider Vinegar, 3 Tablespoons Coconut Oil and 1/3 cup fresh chopped herbs such as basil, rosemary, thyme, oregano, or marjoram. Let mixture sit in the refrigerator for 1 – 2 hours before cooking.

Option 2 – Mix prepared vegetables of choice in a ziplock bag with ¼ cup fresh lemon juice, 3 Tablespoons of Coconut Oil, 2 Tablespoons fresh honey or pure maple syrup, 1 thinly sliced jalapeno, and ½ teaspoon of sea salt. Let mixture sit in the refrigerator for 1 -2 hours before cooking.

Option 3 – Mix prepared vegetables of choice in a ziplock bag with ¼ cup red wine vinegar, 3 Tablespoons of Coconut Oil, ½ teaspoon Smoked Paprika, ½ teaspoon garlic powder, ½ teaspoon onion powder, and ½ teaspoon salt. Let mixture sit in the refrigerator for 1 – 2 hours before cooking.

DRINK UP!!

Make sure to get in your fluids!

Acceptable drinks are:

- ✓ Water with Fresh Lemon Slices
- ✓ Water with Apple Cider Vinegar (about 1 Tablespoon per 8 ounces of water)
- ✓ Seltzer Water with Lemon, Lime, or Orange Slices
- ✓ Green Tea
- ✓ Herbal Tea
- ✓ Homemade Vitamin Water – fresh fruit infused water (keep a pitcher in the fridge filled with water, fresh fruit slices, and herbs of choice)

SUPPLEMENT UP!!

Recommended Dietary Supplements:
1. Daily Essential Multi-Vitamin
2. Protein Powder
3. Powdered Greens
4. Quality Probiotics
5. Quality Omega-3 Fish Oil
6. Vitamin D3

USE CODE: GETLEAN30 for 30% OFF to Stock Up on the above supplements at Olympian Labs

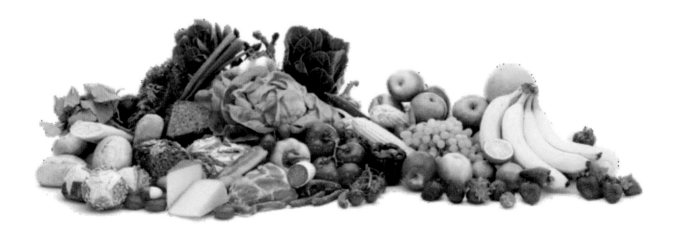

FINAL TIPS AND REMINDERS FOR STAYING HEALTHY AND LEAN:

✓ If it has a large advertising budget, don't eat it. (Michael Pollan) So, basically avoid all processed foods.

✓ Make a weekly Meal Plan and shop according to what you need for it so you have everything on hand.

✓ Shop only the perimeter of your grocery store. The aisles are where all the junk is (expect maybe tea, frozen veggies/lean meats and oatmeal).

✓ Never shop on an empty stomach. Write your list before you go, and stick to it.

✓ Make double, even triple, batches of everything you cook. Then freeze the extras so you can just thaw and warm for your busy mornings and evenings.

✓ Keep cut and prepped fresh vegetables and fruit in the refrigerator ready for those "snack attacks".

✓ Find out if you have any food sensitivities, then avoid those foods completely. It's tough, but you'll feel so much better!

✓ Drink water. A lot of it. Every day.

✓ Move/sweat daily. It does not take a lot of time to get in an amazing fat-burning interval workout.

✓ Take the time to get to know what your body really needs. Every person is unique.

✓ Be kind enough to your body to exclude the foods that your body does not like or has negative reactions to.

✓ Health is a state of mind. If you change your mind and the way you think, you'll change your body too.

✓ Try and plant a small garden. Grow a few things in pots. Let the kids help. Fresh greens and herbs are so simple to grow and you will love being able to go out and grab what you need whenever you need it.

✓ This is a journey. Take it a step at a time.

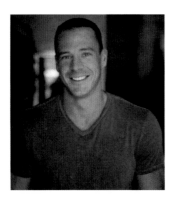

Jeremy Scott is a **certified fitness professional and nutrition specialist** and the creator of **Jeremy Scott Fitness** (www.jeremyscottfitness.com) in Scottsdale, AZ. He was recently voted one of the TOP 50 Hottest Trainers in America by Shape Magazine in 2013 & 2014, in addition to being a nationally published author and contributing writer to various fitness publications. Jeremy is a Reebok One Ambassador & Elite Contributor for Fitfluential. His unique training style and nutrition protocols have helped thousands of people all across America get into and stay in the best shape of their lives. Jeremy is also known for his best selling self-help book. "Make Success Mandatory".

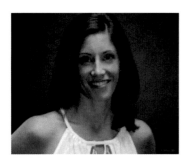

Kim Maes, CNC, AADP known as the Allergy Free Food Coach, is a Certified Nutrition Consultant and Certified in the Practical Application of Food Allergy Guidelines. She is also the creator of the award-winning Cook It Allergy Free iPhone and iPad Apps and the Cook It Allergy Free website (www.cookitallergyfree.com). She is Associate Editor for the top-selling Simply...Gluten-Free Magazine and has been featured in numerous other leading magazines and websites. She focuses on teaching immune-boosting nutrition to improve life with Autism, AD/HD, Food Allergies, Leaky Gut, and more. She offers both personal and online nutrition coaching with customized programs that include meal plans, grocery lists, supplement guidance, cookbooks, and unlimited support for her clients. She teaches them how to feel more confident, more in control, and less overwhelmed about their new path to health.

To learn more about fitness, nutrition, and how to STAY lean and healthy...

You can visit Jeremy Scott at: www.jeremyscottfitness.com

You can visit Kim Maes at: www.cookitallergyfree.com

Made in the USA
San Bernardino, CA
20 January 2020

63392542R00024